GOOD VIBES
COLORING BOOK

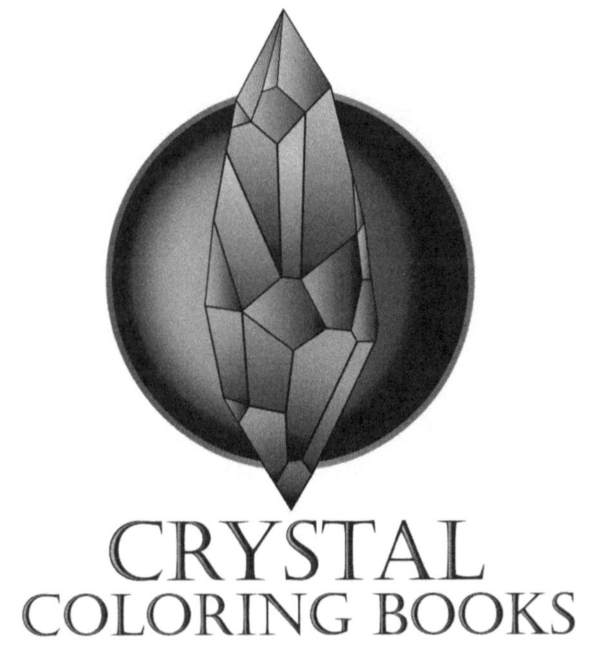

CRYSTAL
COLORING BOOKS

ISBN-13: 978-1986178884
ISBN-10: 1986178889

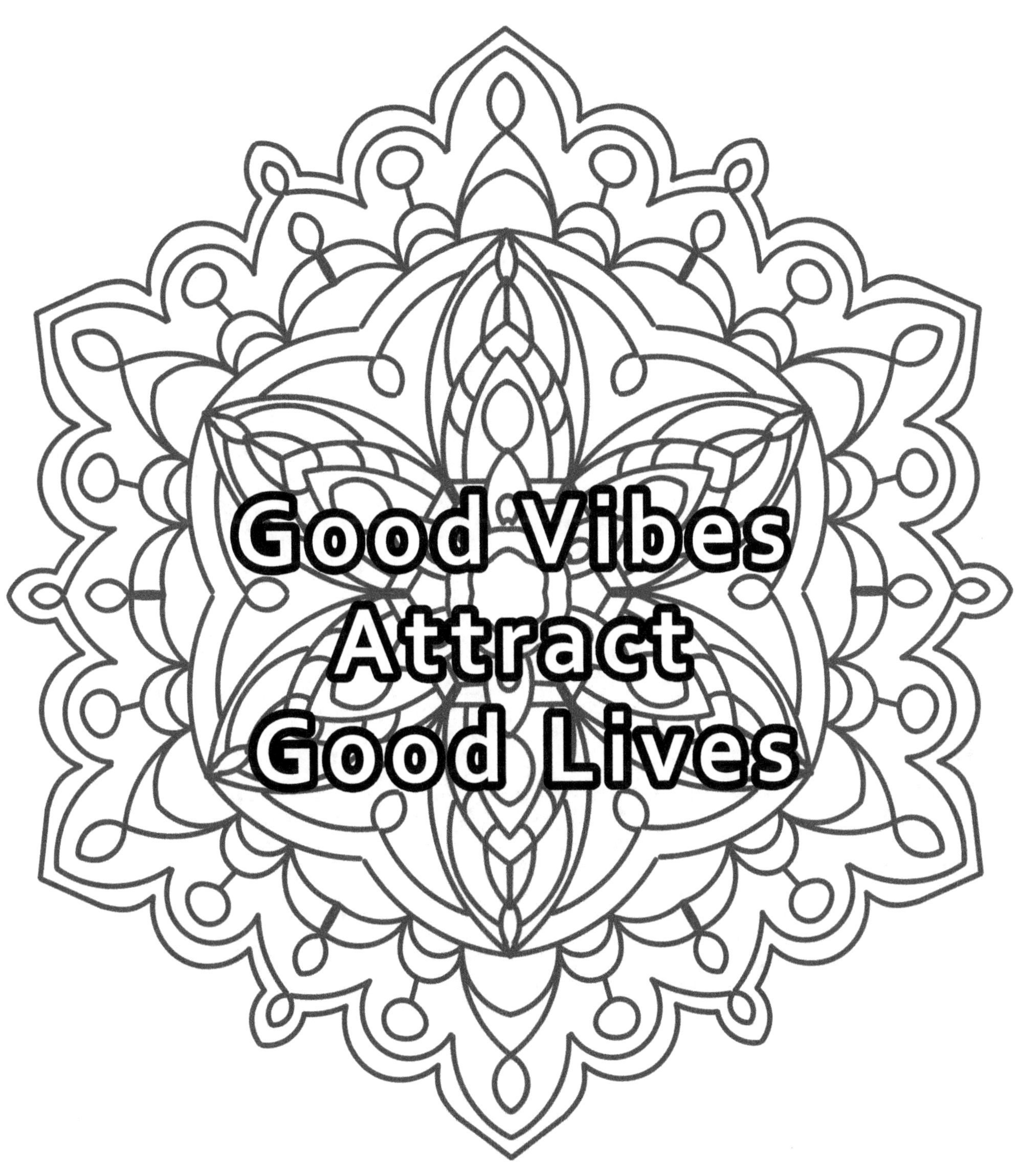

Good Vibes
Attract
Good Lives

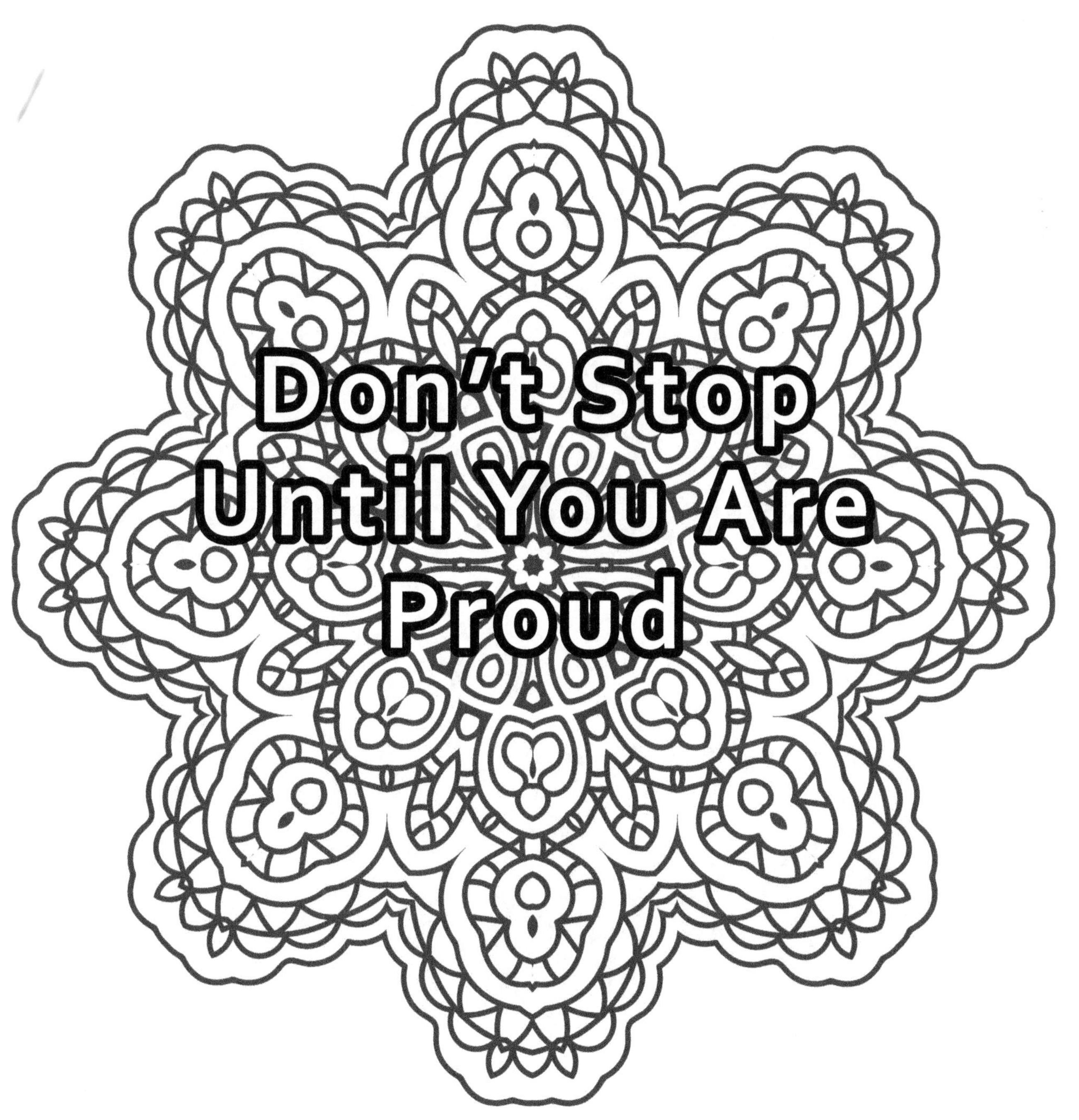

Don't Stop
Until You Are
Proud

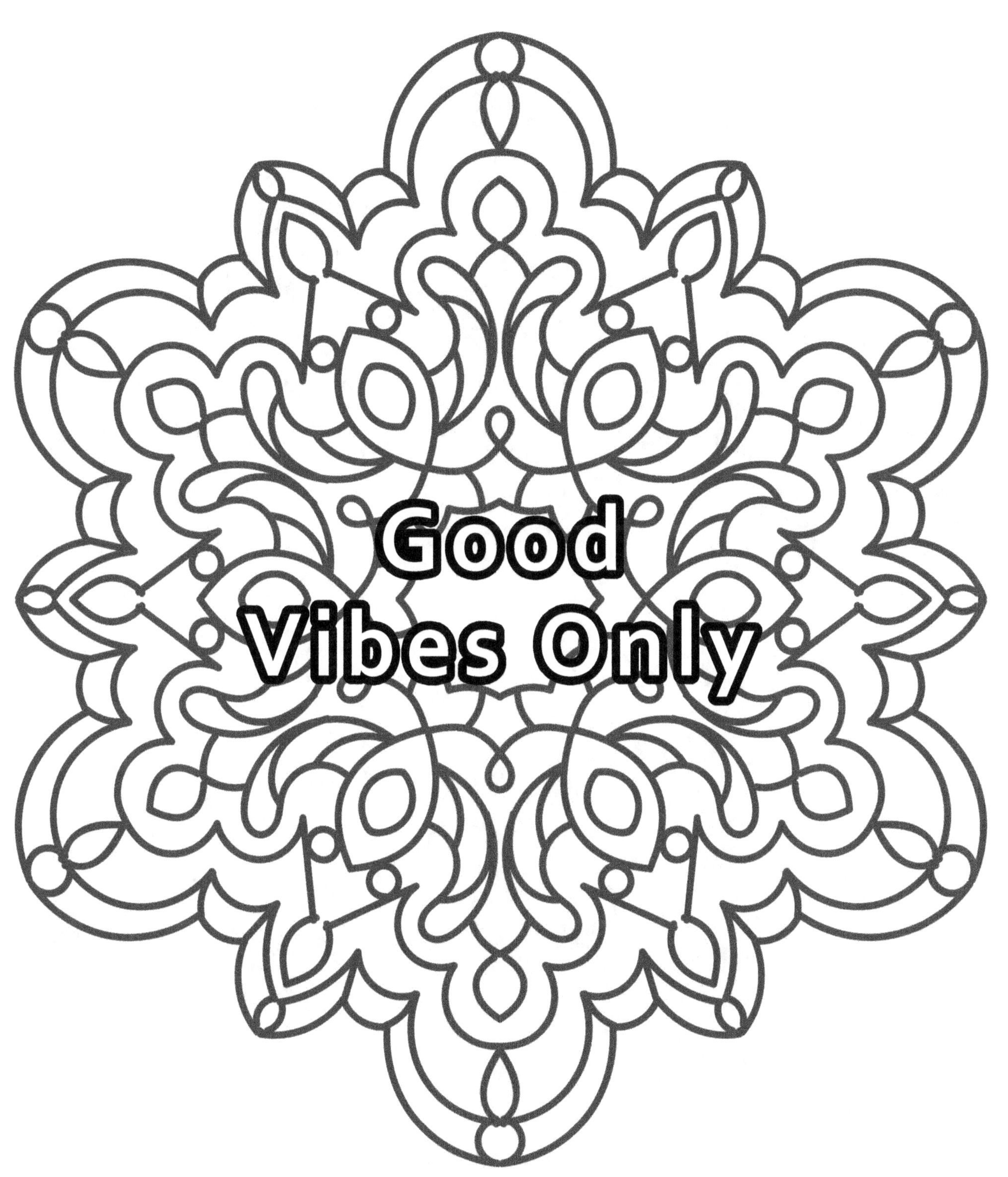
Good
Vibes Only

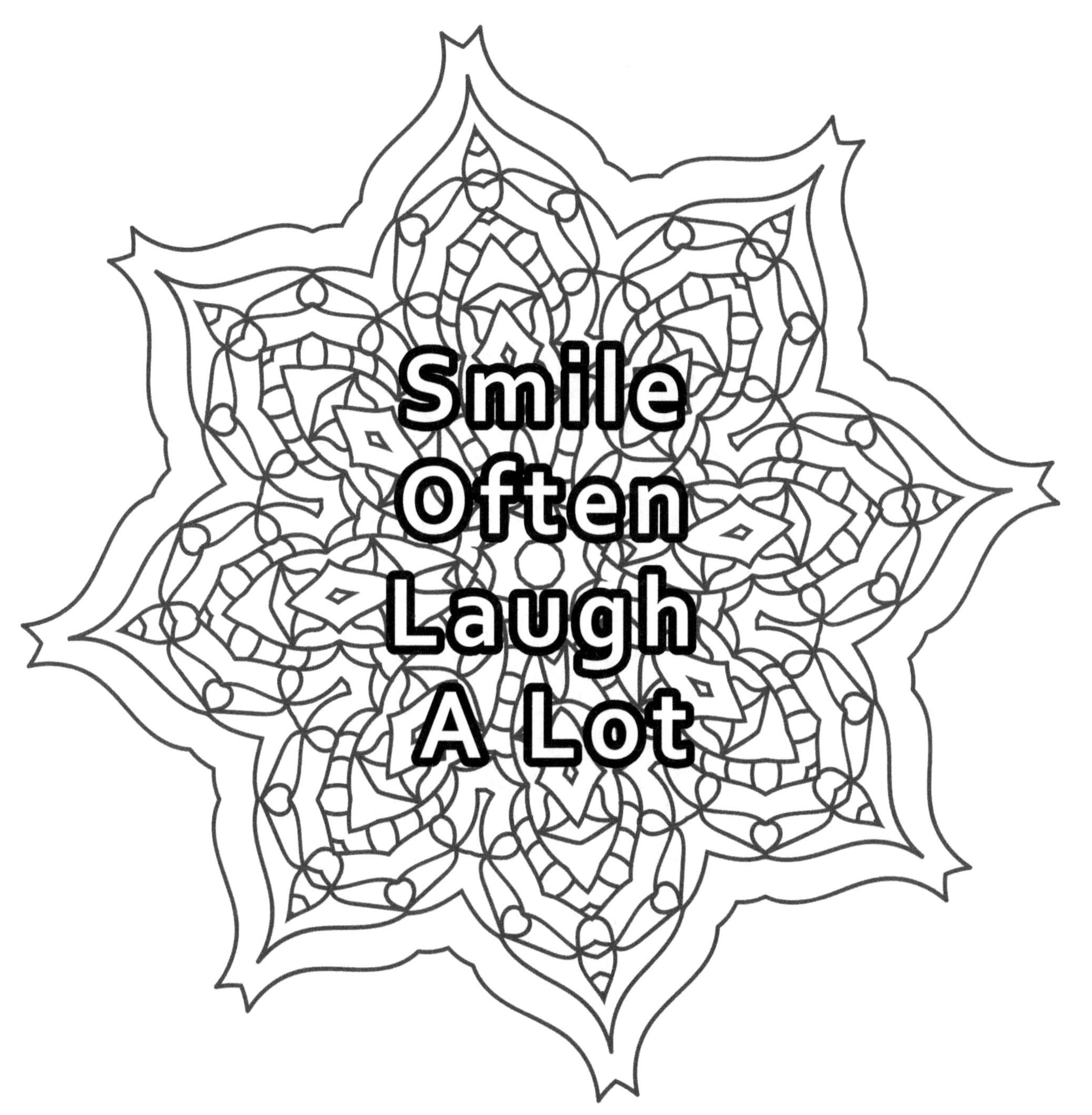

Smile
Often
Laugh
A Lot

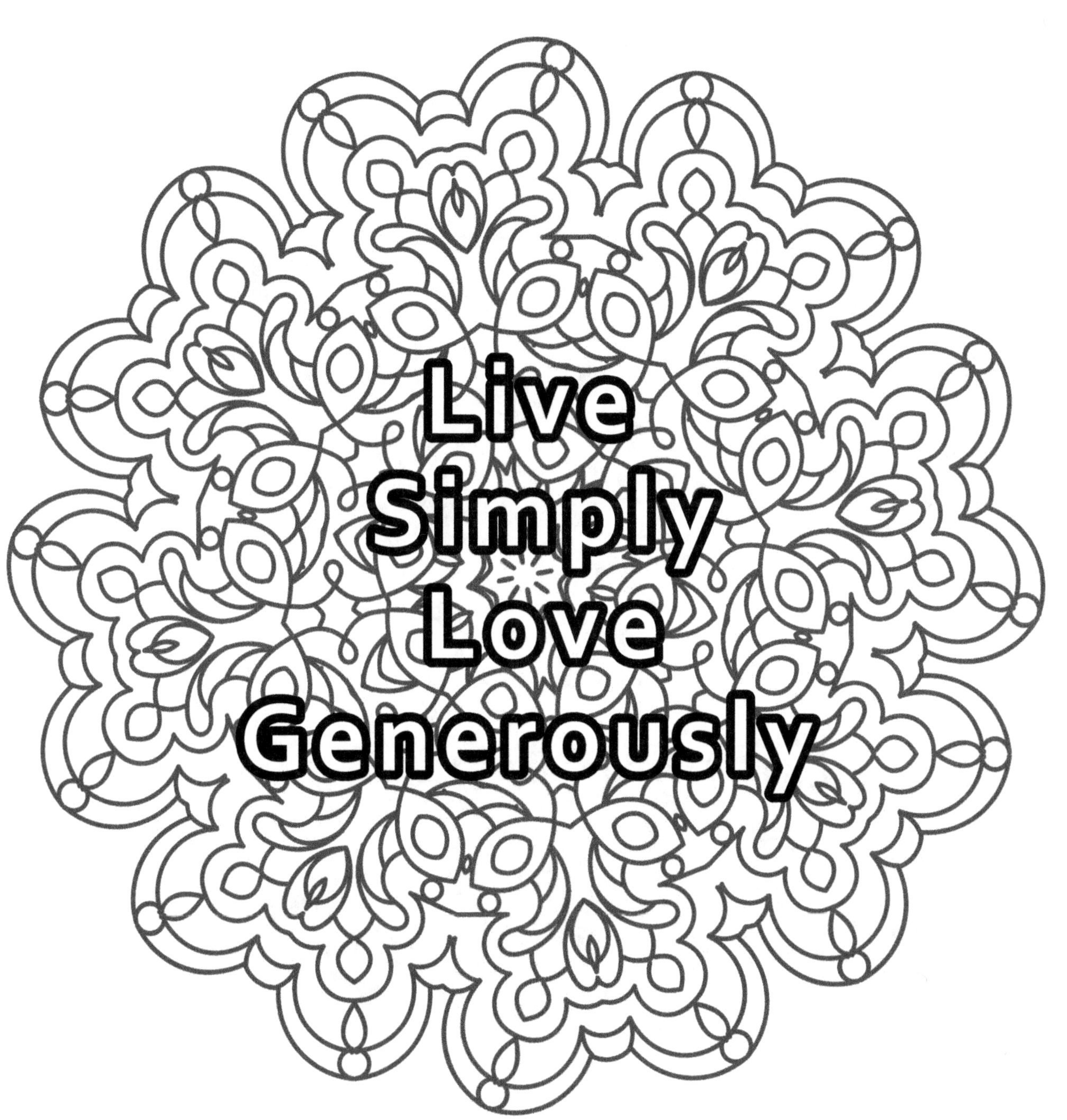
Live
Simply
Love
Generously

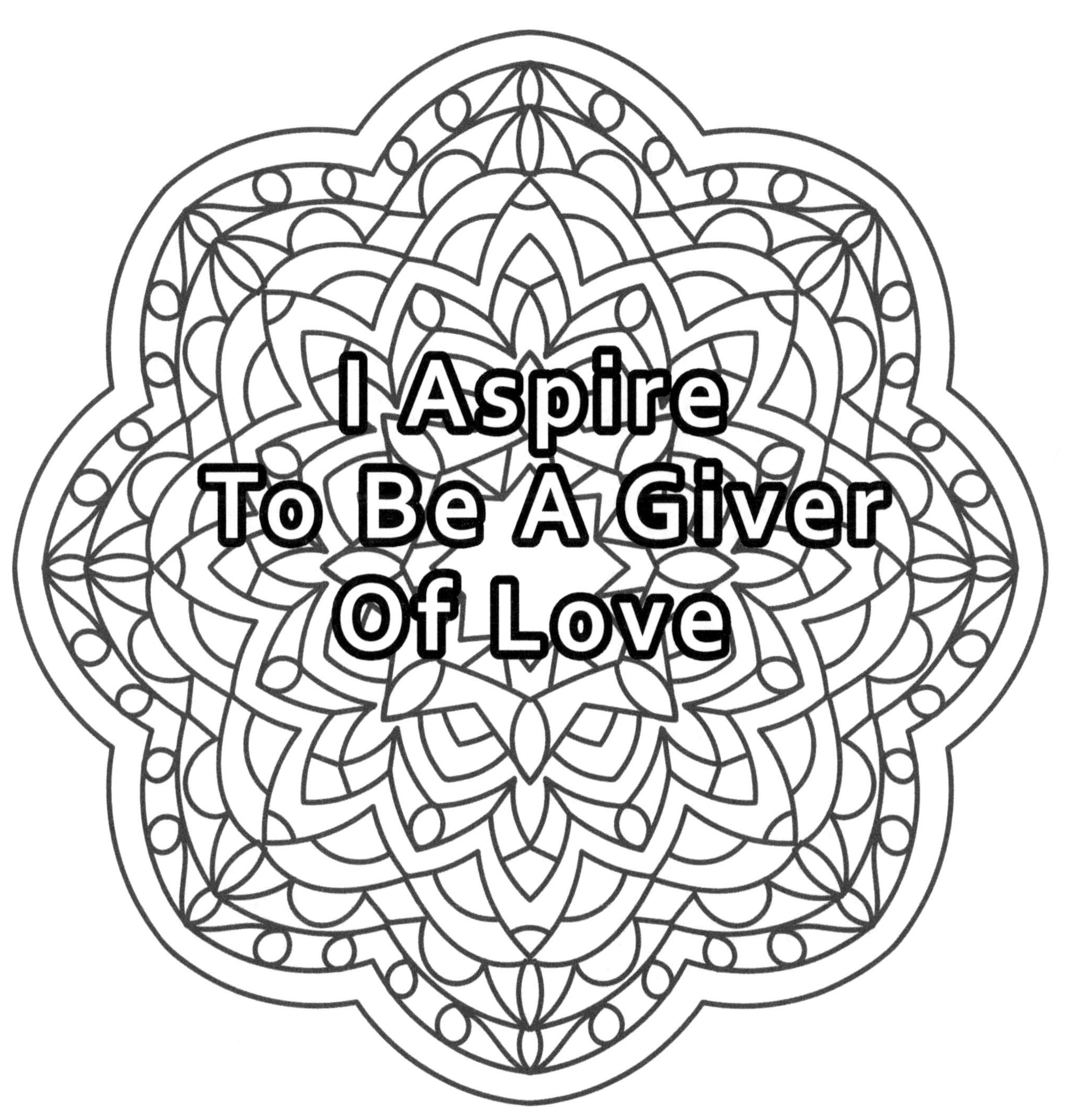
I Aspire
To Be A Giver
Of Love

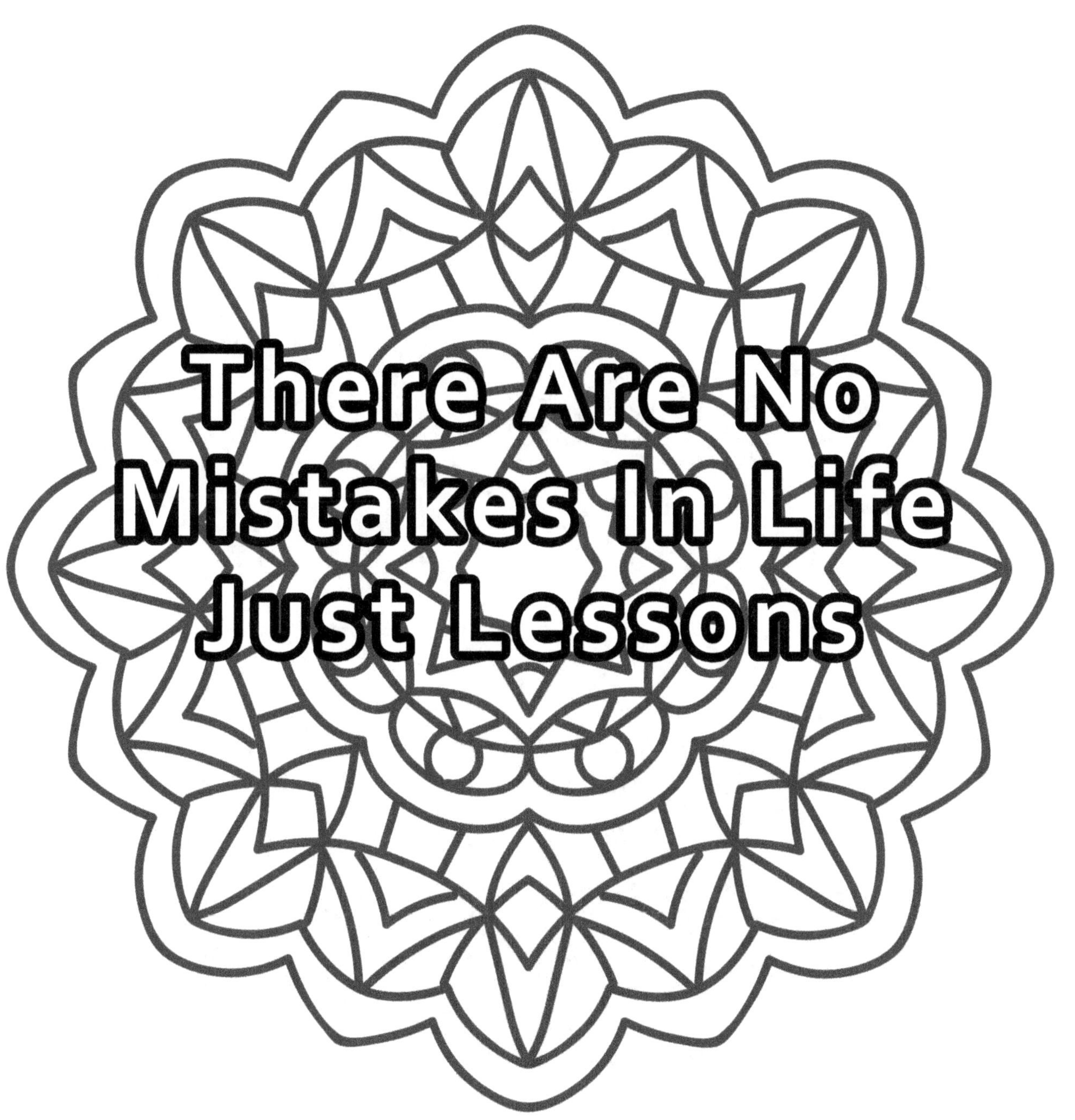
There Are No
Mistakes In Life
Just Lessons

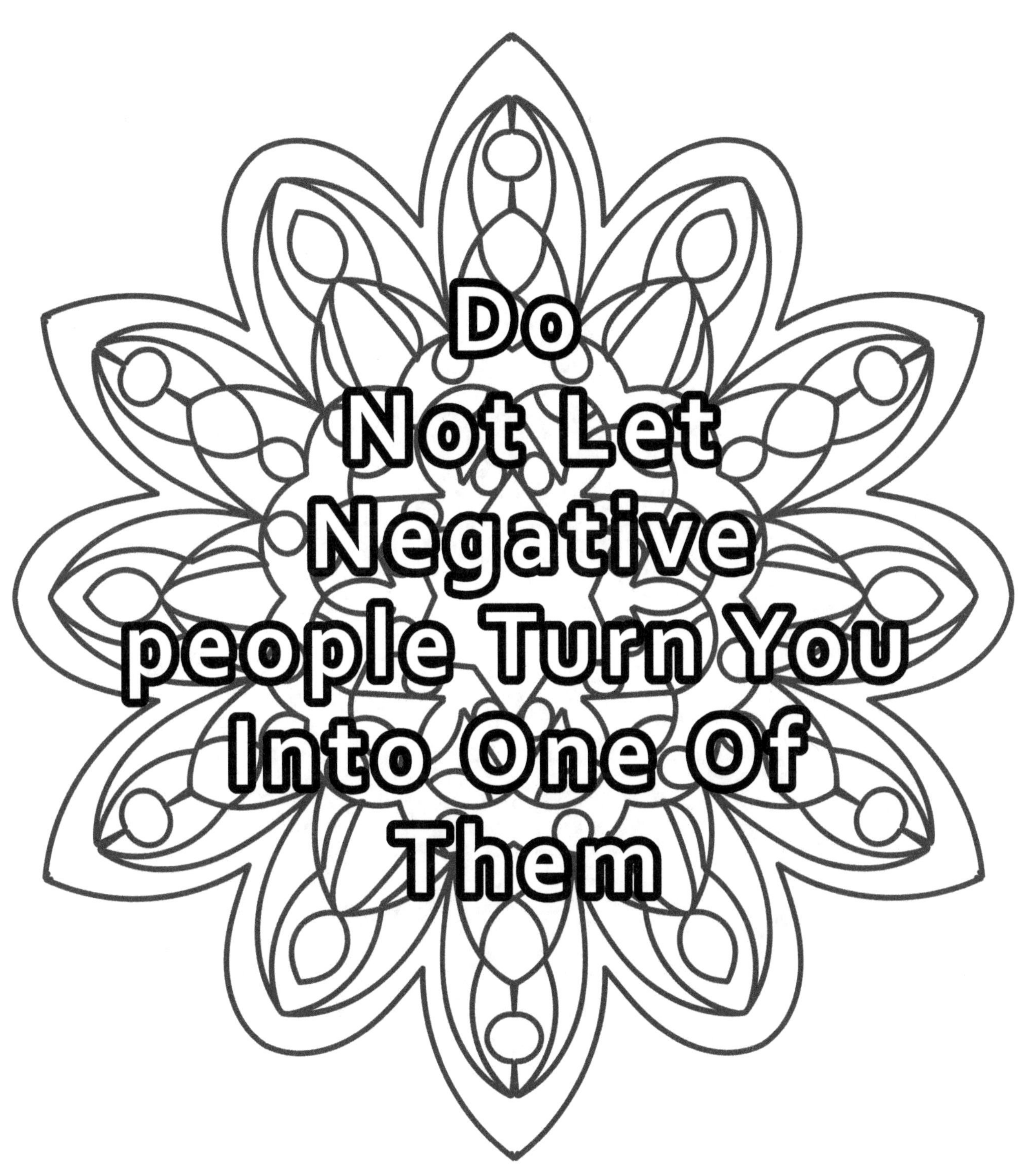
Do
Not Let
Negative
people Turn You
Into One Of
Them

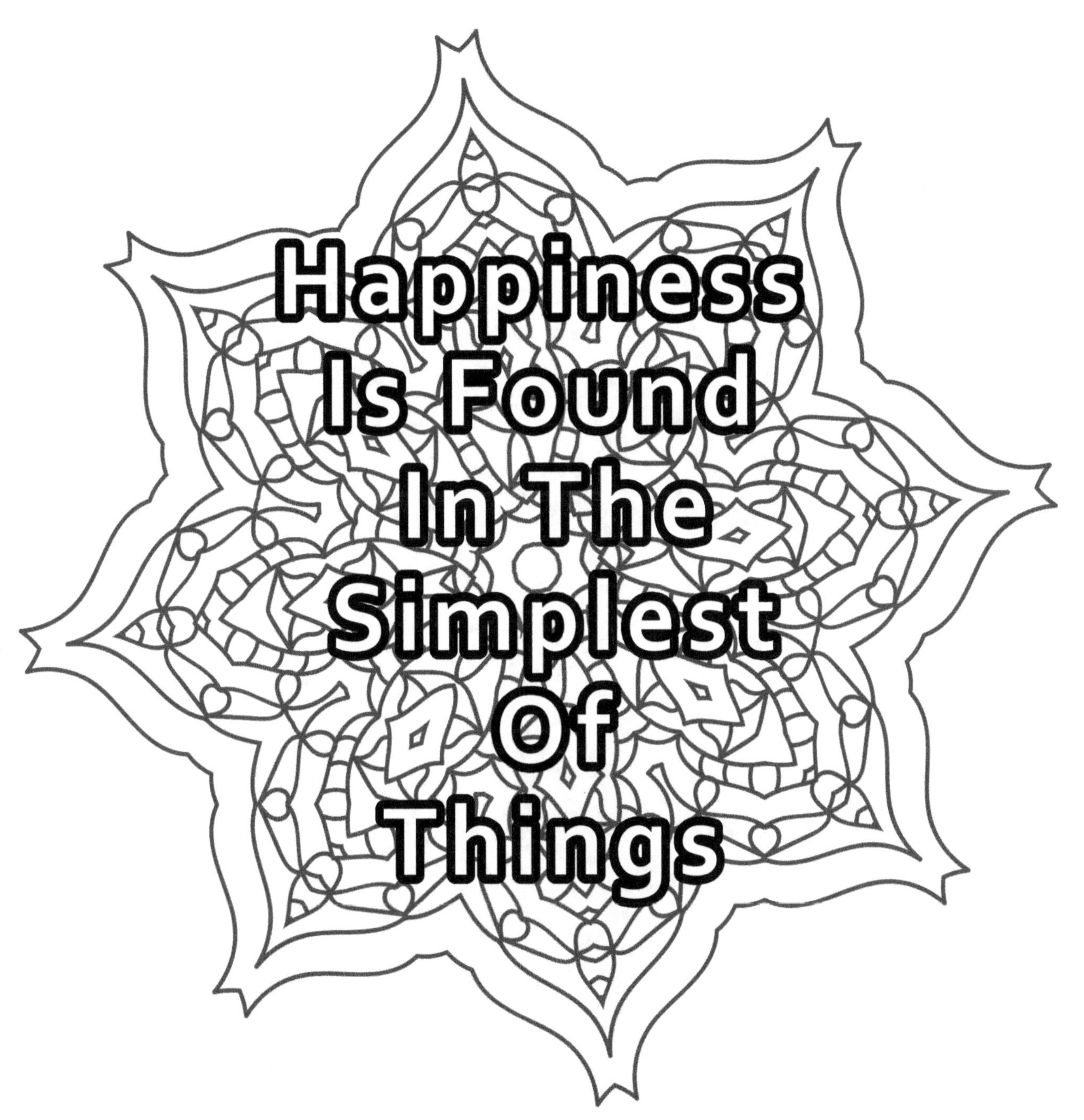

Happiness
Is Found
In The
Simplest
Of
Things

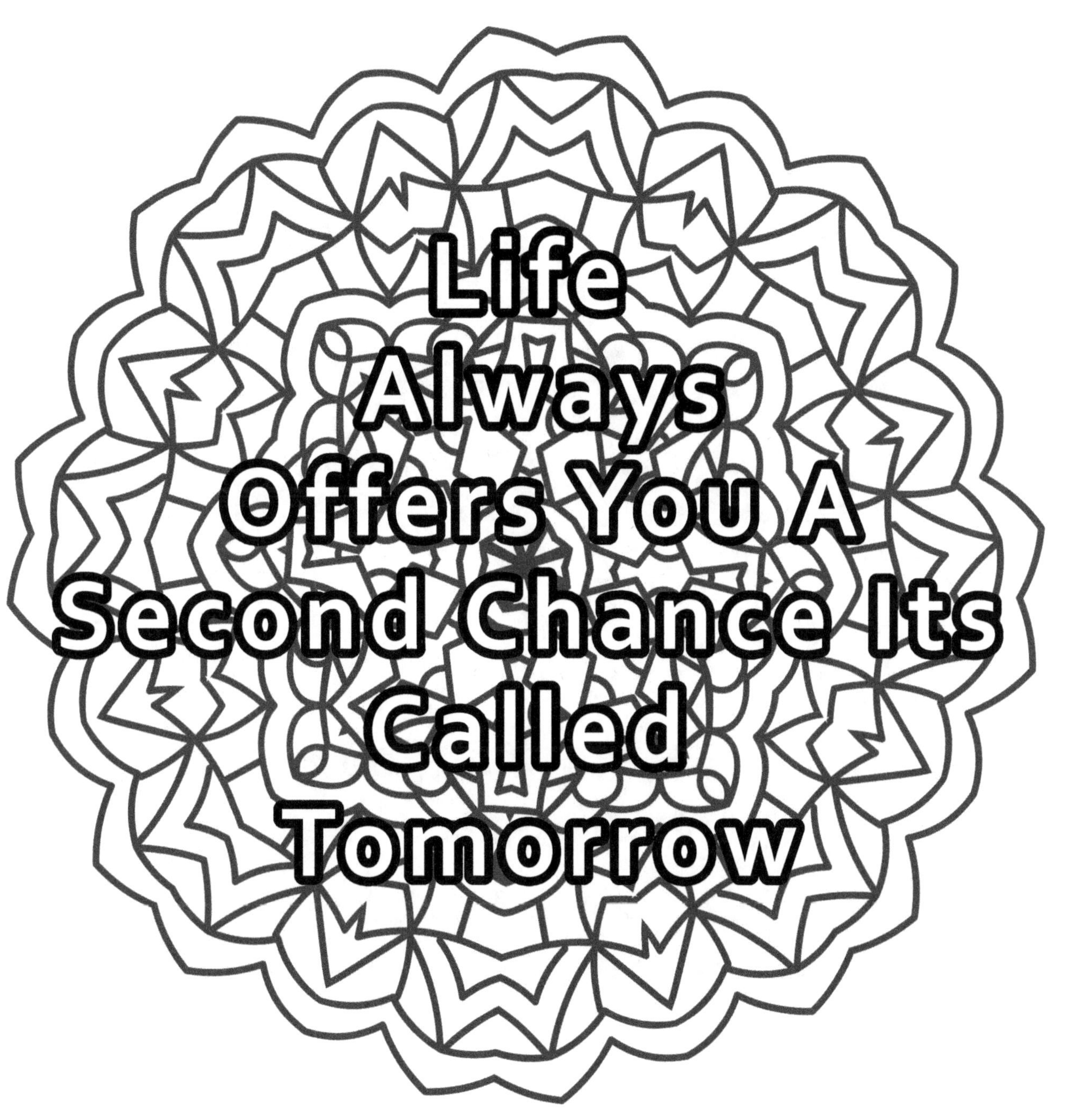

Life
Always
Offers You A
Second Chance Its
Called
Tomorrow

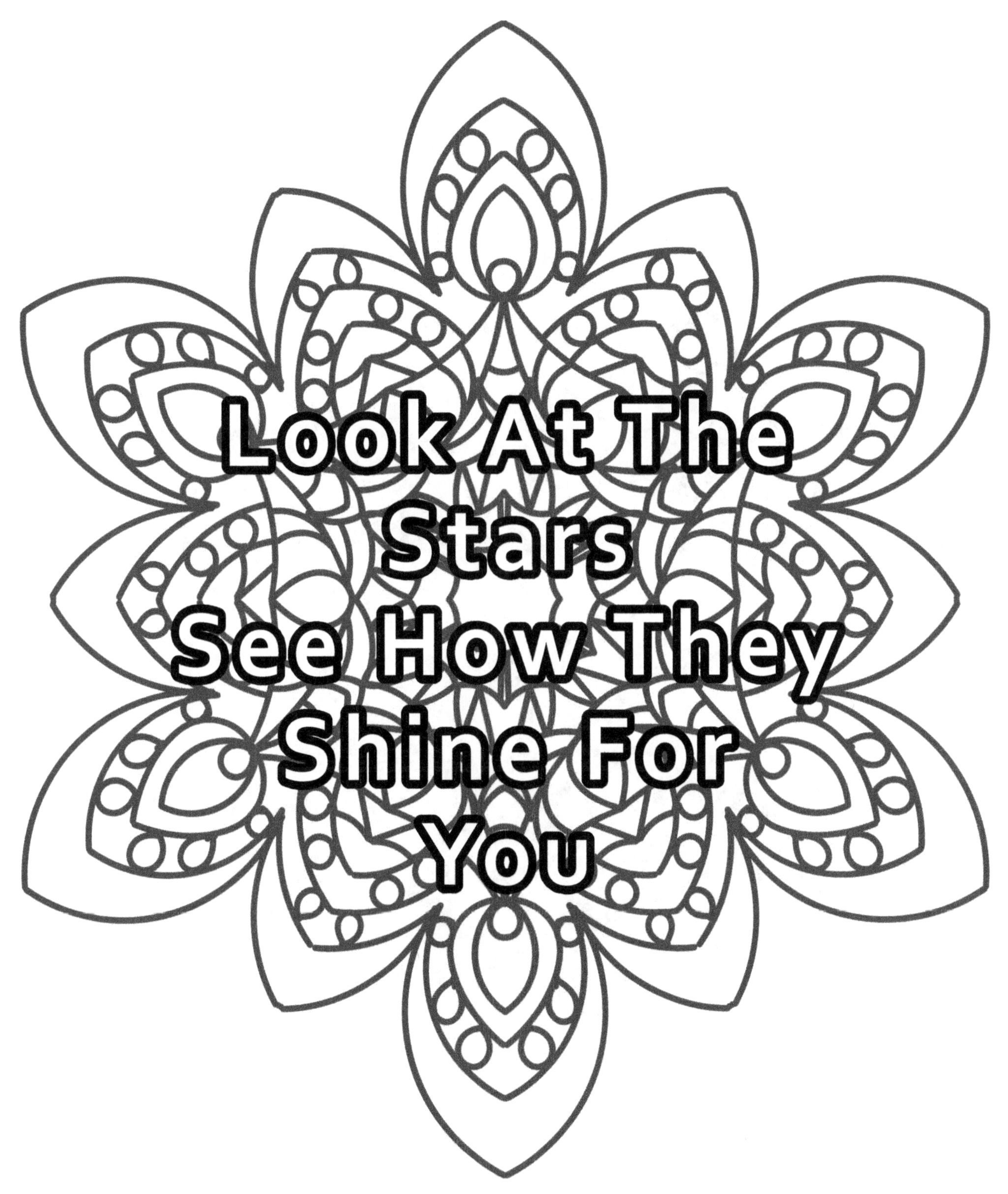
Look At The
Stars
See How They
Shine For
You

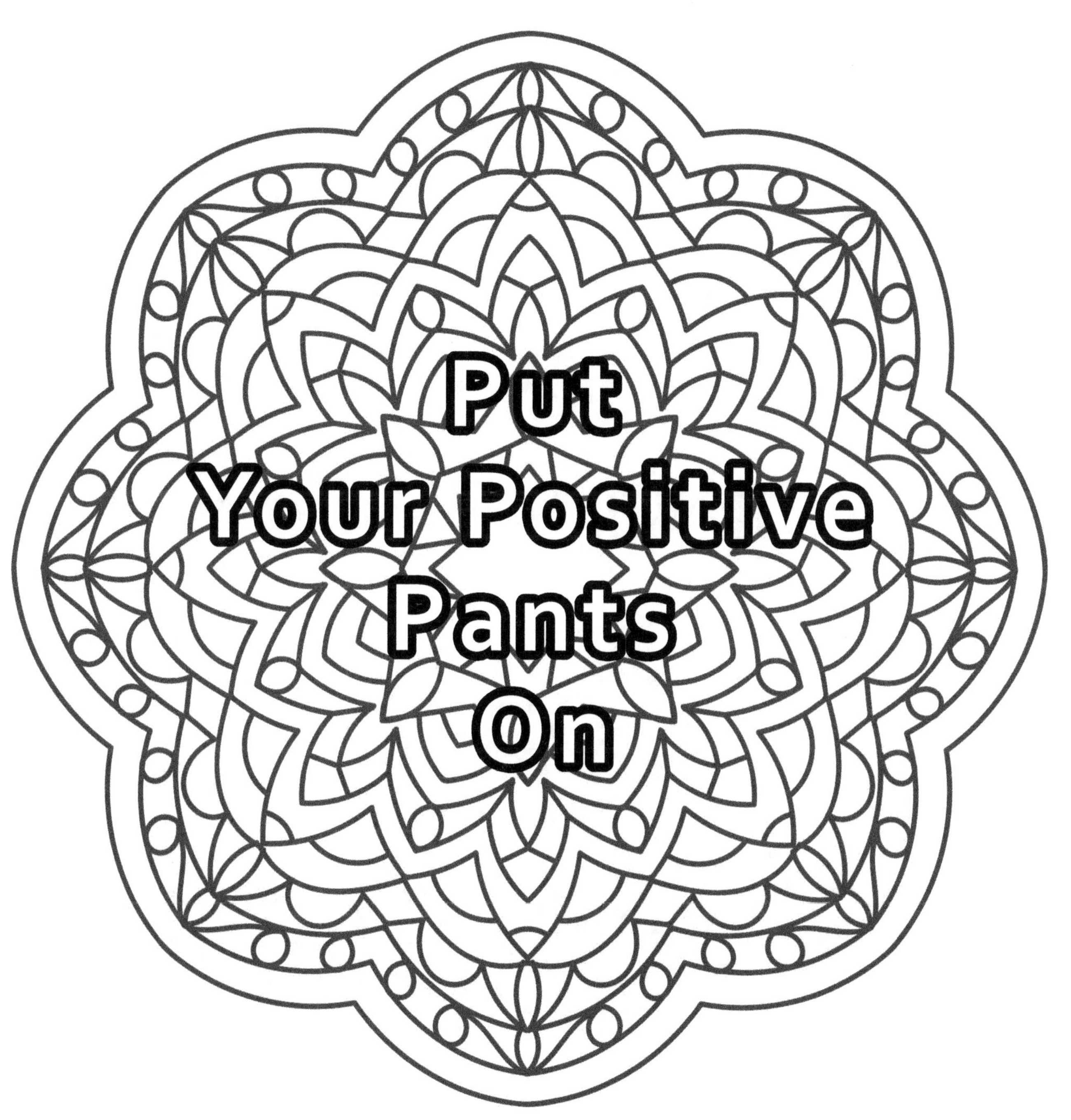
Put
Your Positive
Pants
On

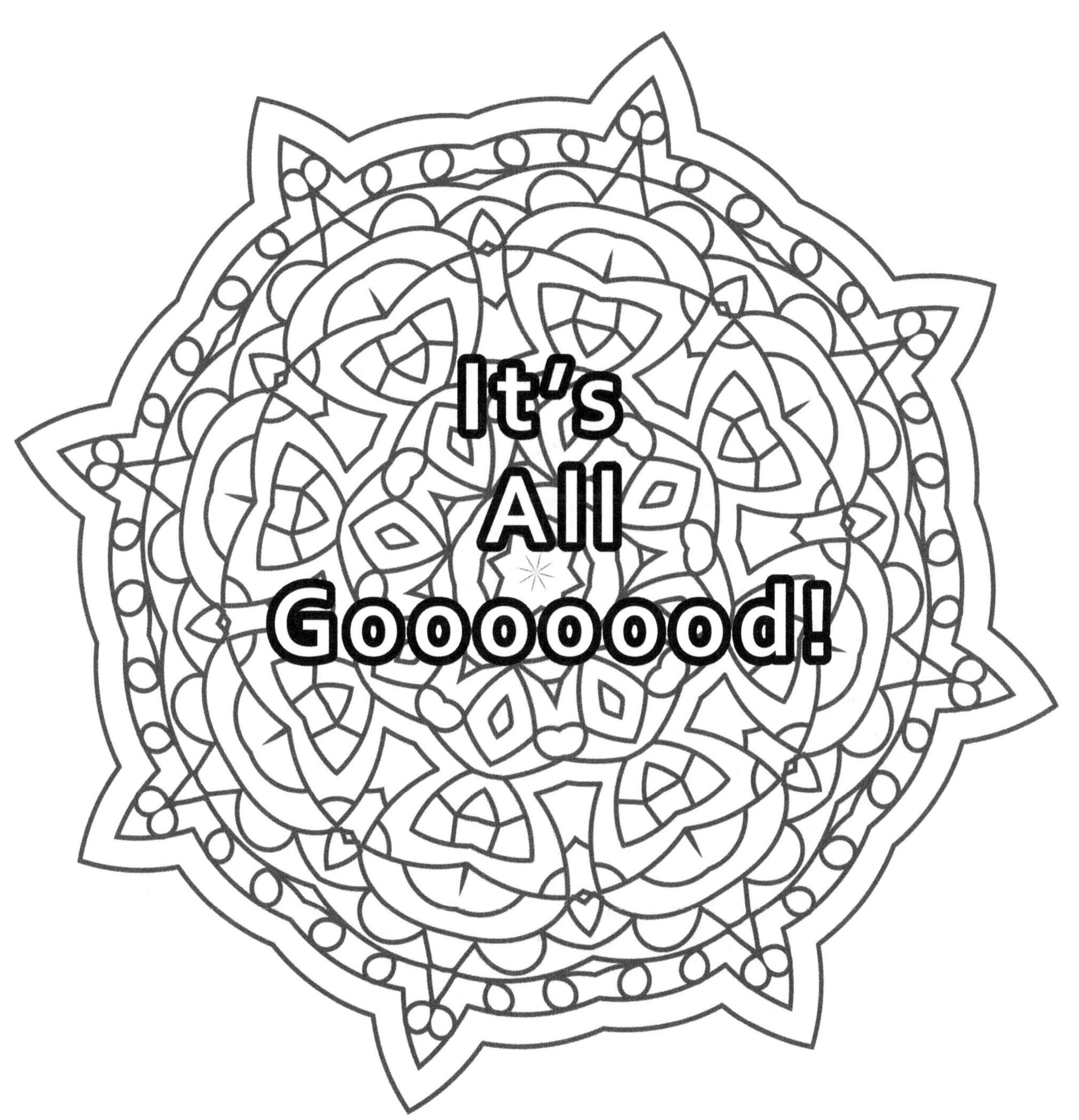
It's
All
Gooooood!

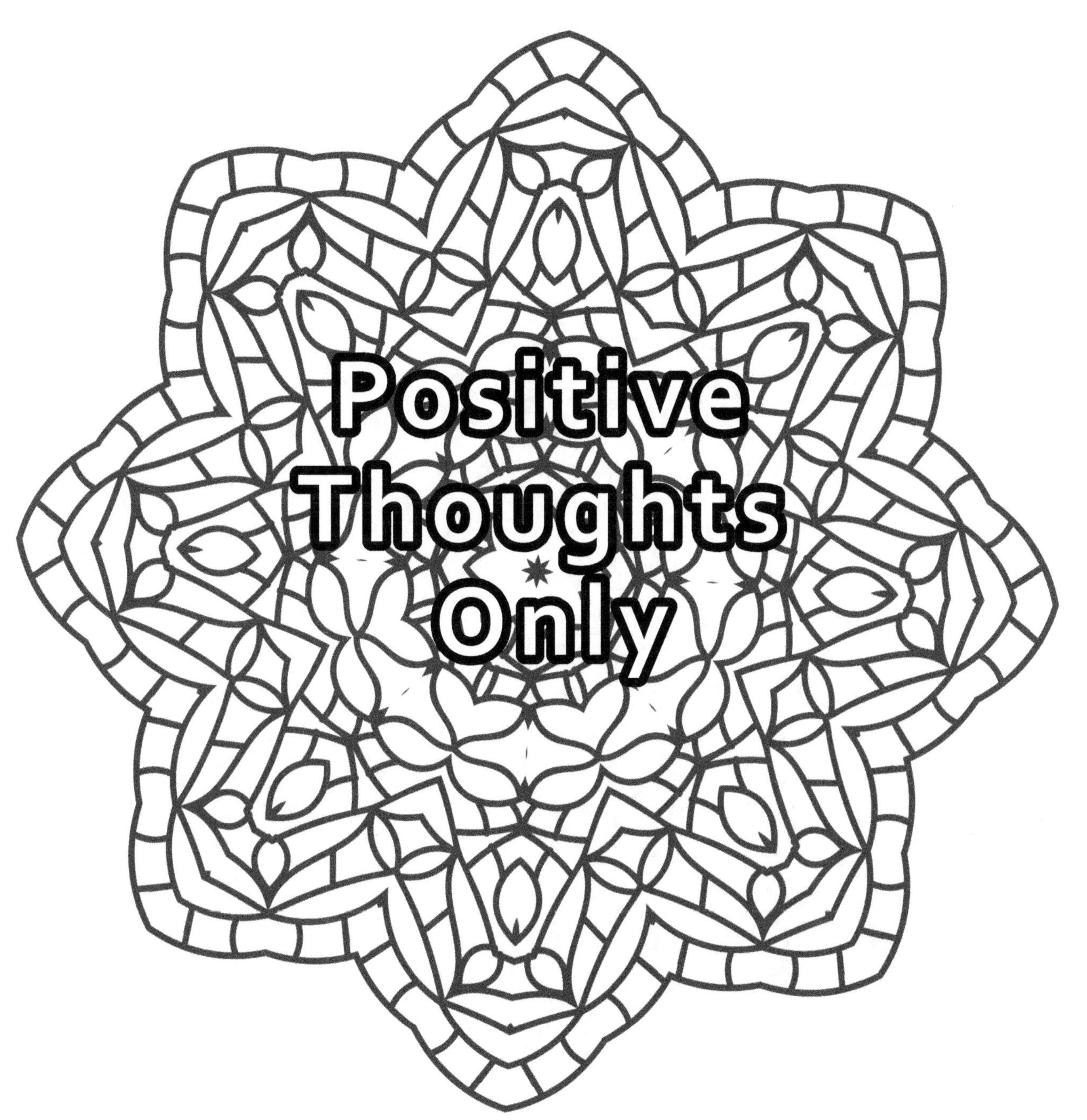
Positive
Thoughts
Only

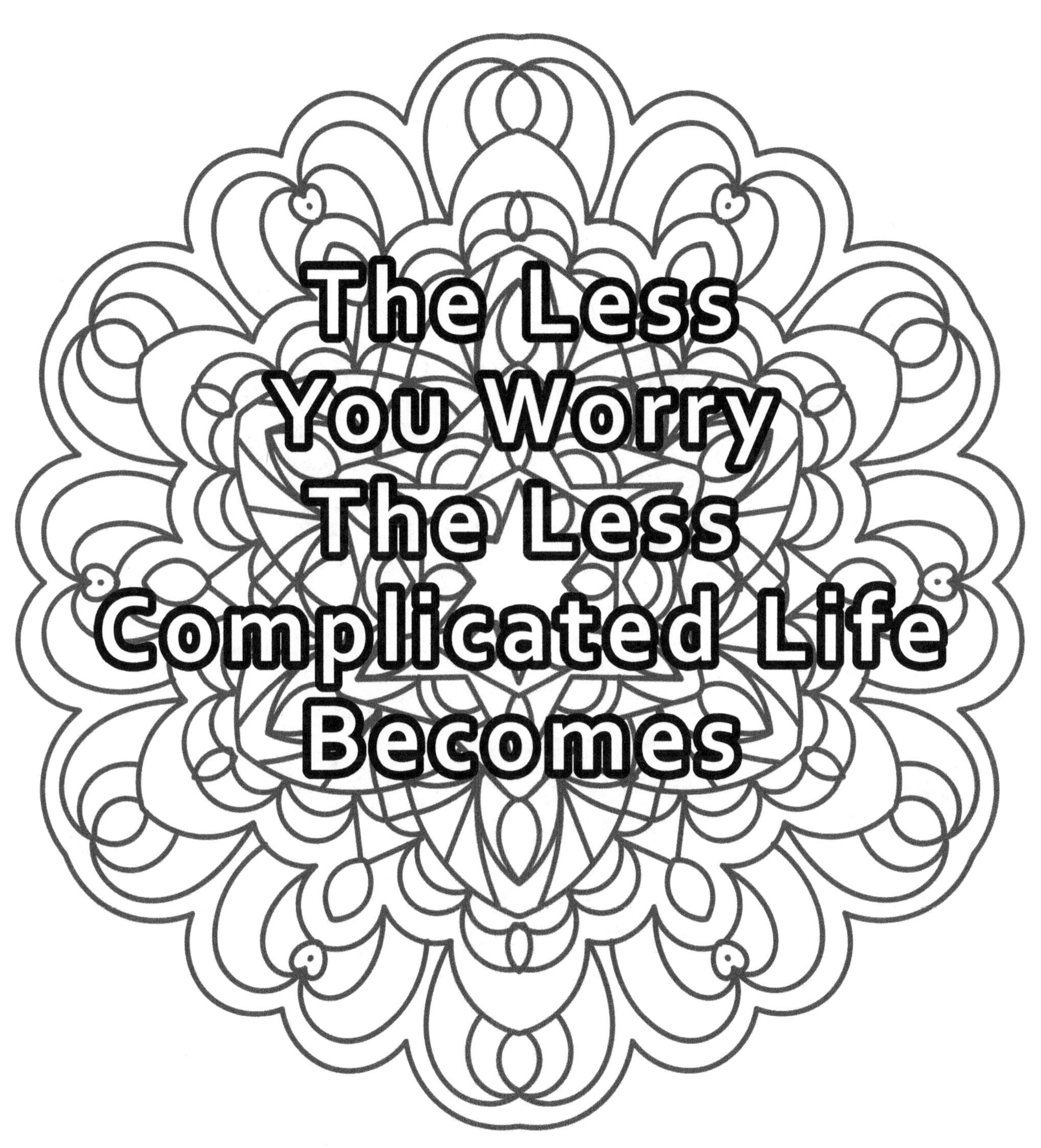

The Less
You Worry
The Less
Complicated Life
Becomes

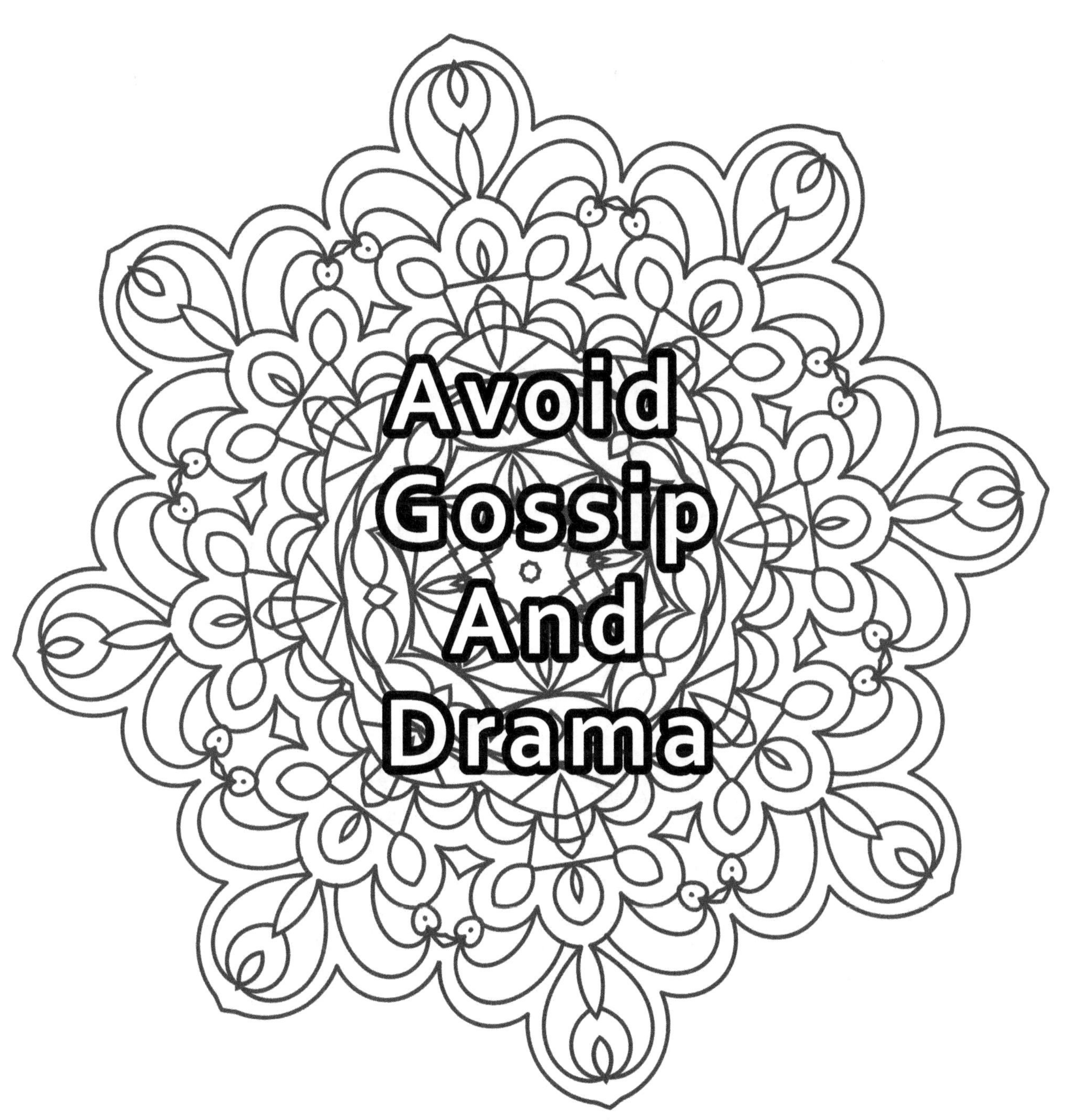

Avoid
Gossip
And
Drama

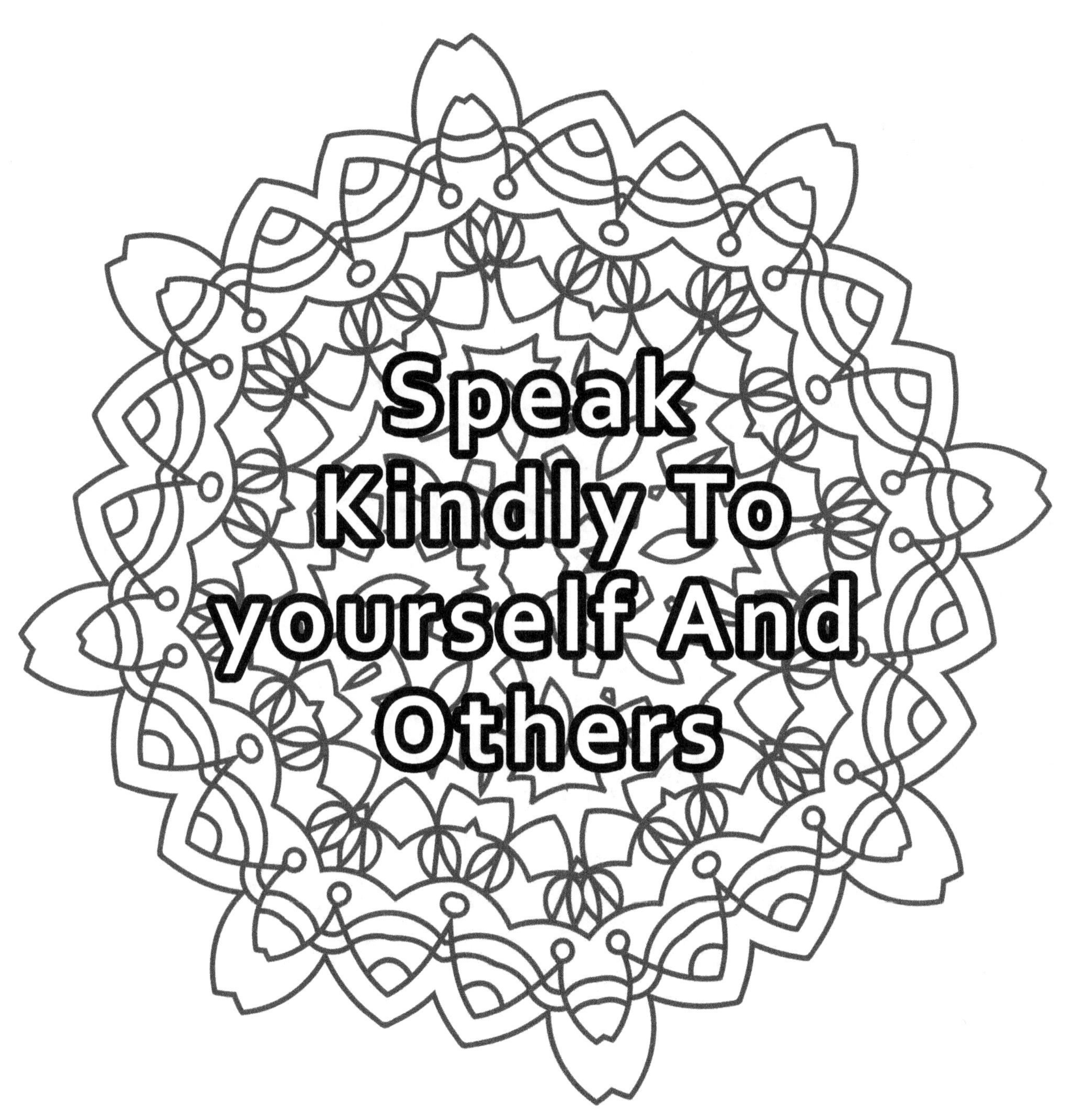
Speak
Kindly To
yourself And
Others

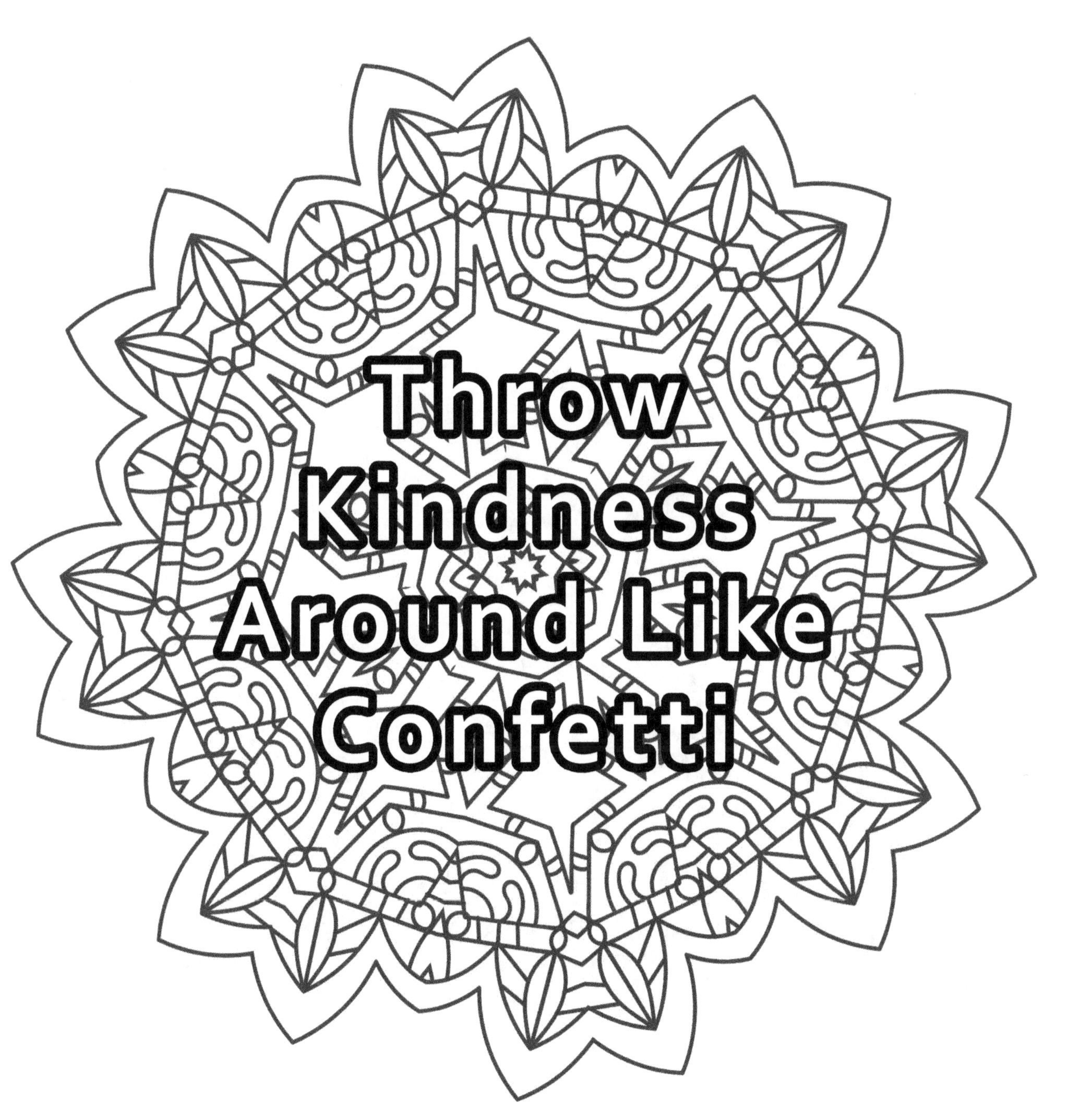

Throw
Kindness
Around Like
Confetti

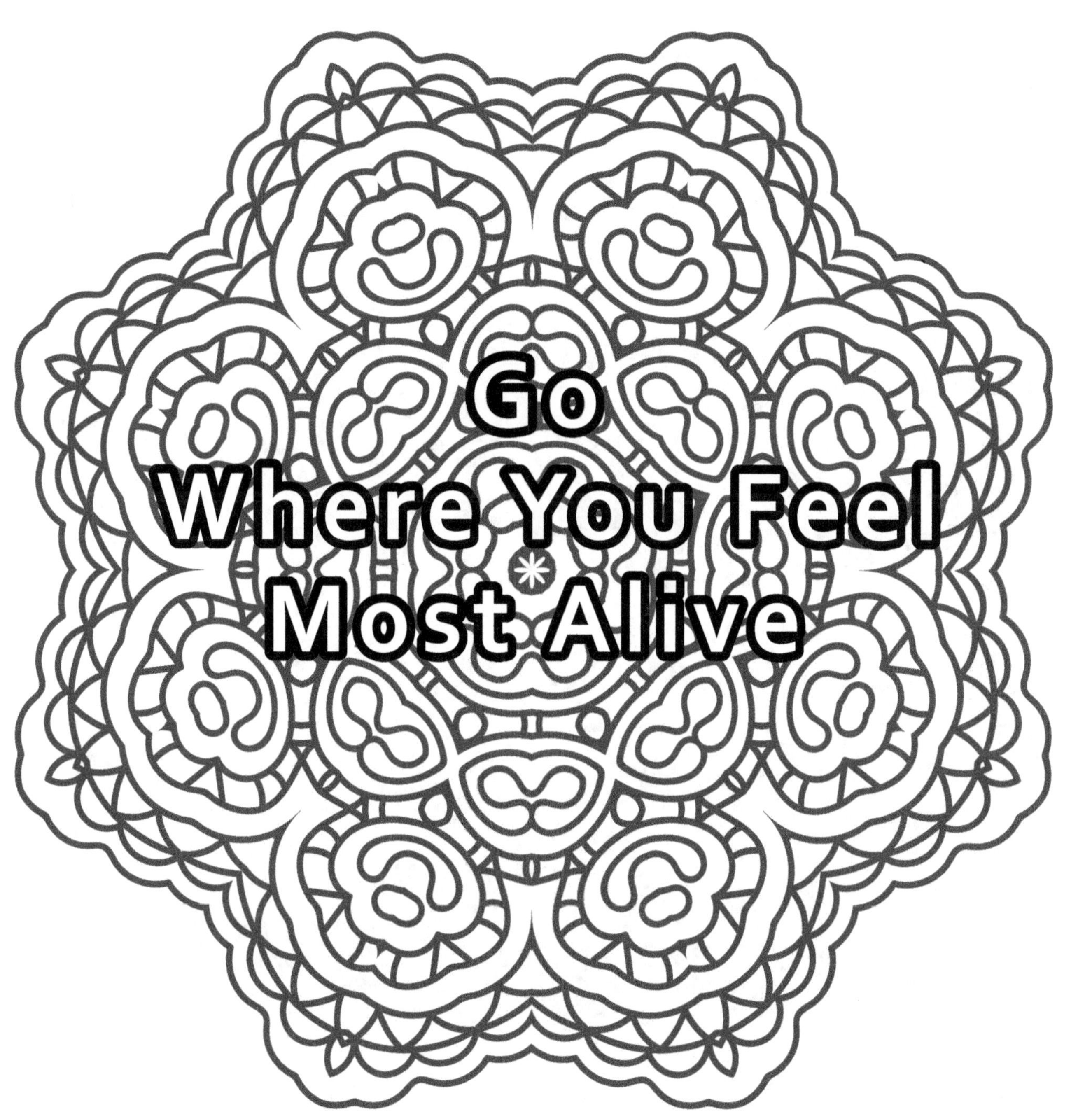
Go
Where You Feel
Most Alive

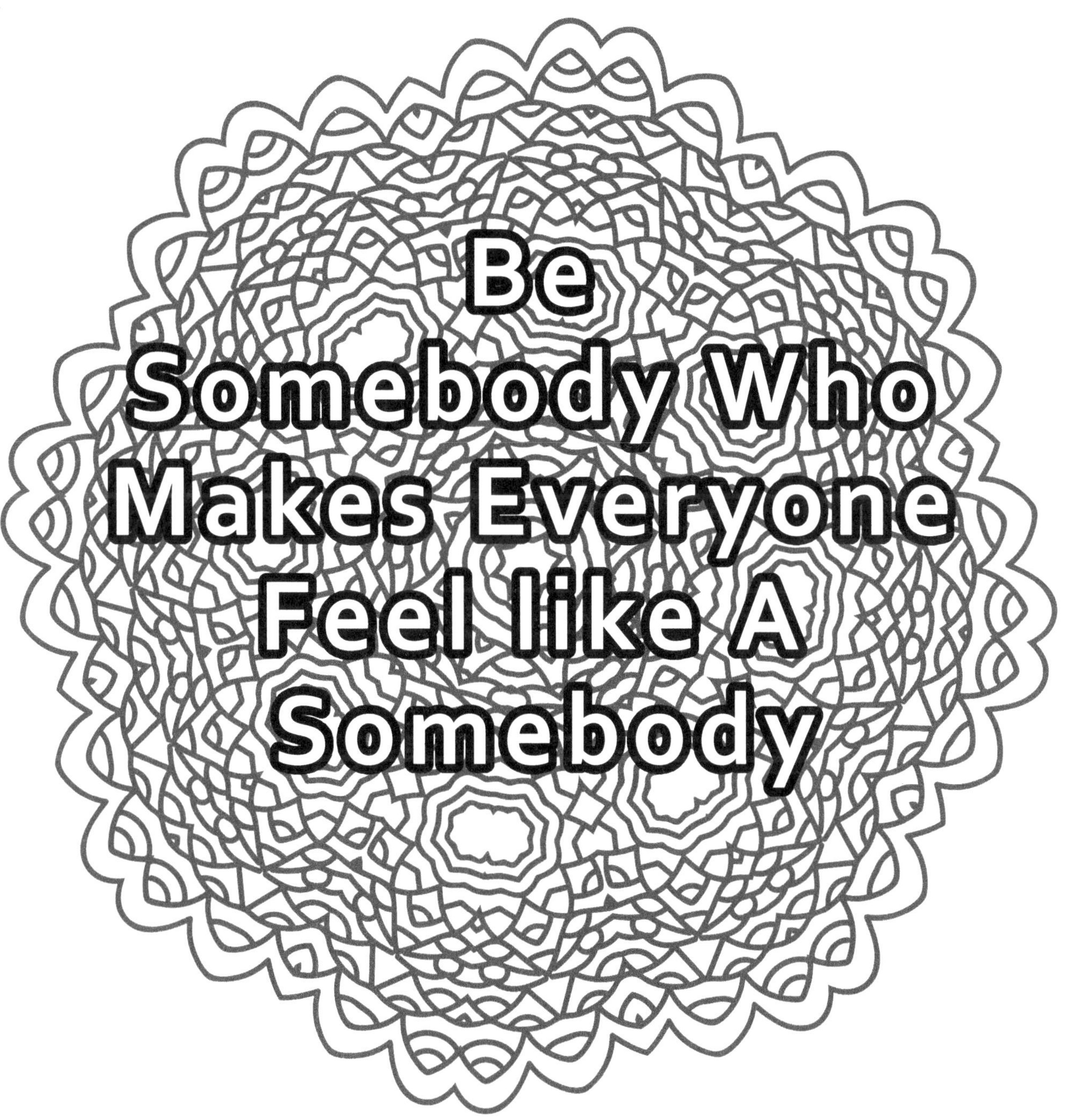

Be
Somebody Who
Makes Everyone
Feel like A
Somebody

COLOR TEST PAGE

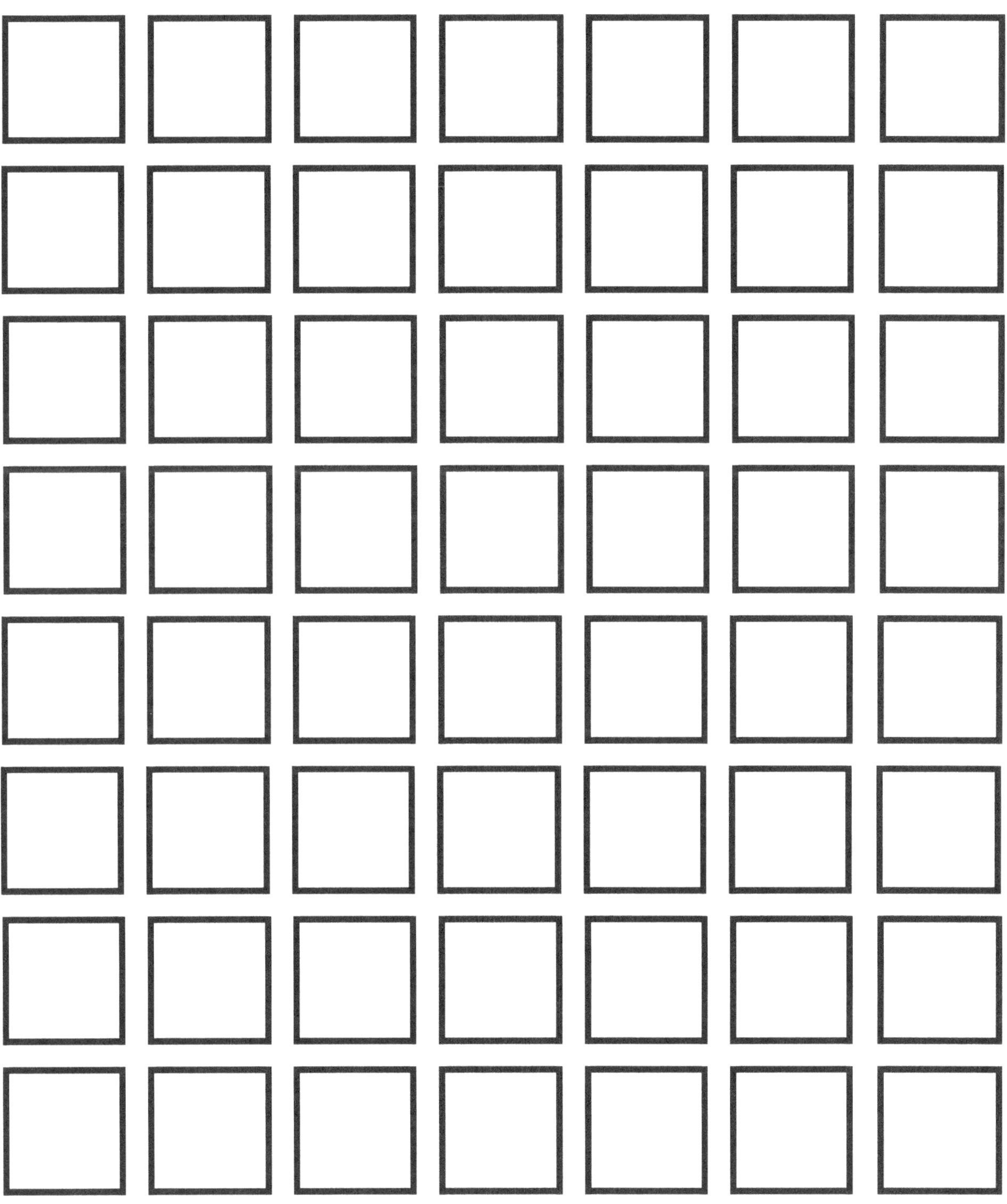